EAT OR BE EATEN

Between The Hidden Dangers of Fad Diets and Quick Fixes

OLOJO CHRISTIANA

INTRODUCTION

In this digital social media-driven era where information is at every touch of a button, people are getting obsessed with having the 'perfect' body. "UNHEALTHY DIETING: Between The Hidden Dangers of Fad Diets and Quick Fixes" sets out to unravel the many layers of diet culture and to bring forth those dangers that usually are not considered while relentlessly chasing fast results.

Every day, millions of people are bombarded by the newest and greatest fad diets that promise miraculous transformations. From juice cleanses to ketogenic regimens, these quick fixes often prioritize immediate weight loss over long-term health, leading many down a path fraught with nutritional deficiencies, disordered eating, and emotional turmoil. The allure of rapid results is intoxicating, but the hidden costs are rarely discussed.

I am going to delve deeply into the dieting landscape, investigating which psychological, social, and physiological factors link to unhealthy eating behaviors. We will investigate nutritional science, the power of societal pressure, and the role of media in shaping our views on health and beauty. It is through an understanding of such influences that we are able to begin to break down some of the myths about dieting and develop a much healthier relationship with food.

As we journey through this together, let me lead you to take a reflection of your personal experiences about dieting. Think about what motivated you toward such a decision and what effects those decisions have brought into your physical and mental health. By cultivating awareness and compassion, we will be able to empower ourselves to make informed decisions that prioritize our overall well-being.

Welcome to "UNHEALTHY DIETING." Together, let's navigate the complexities of dieting culture and uncover a path toward lasting health and happiness.

CONTENTS

ACKNOWLEDGMENTS

I would like to take this opportunity to express my appreciation to all those who have made the writing of "Unhealthy Dieting: Between The Hidden Dangers of Fad Diets and Quick Fixes" possible.

A word of thanks to one and all-families and friends, for steadfast encouragement and believing in my vision. This means the world to me.

I am also indebted to my mentors and other professionals in the field of health and nutrition, since their insights and expertise have enriched this work so much.

Editors and publishing team, thanks once more for your guidance and effort put into bringing this book to life.

Last but not least, I would like to thank my readers. Their curiosity to know more about how dieting works inspires me each day, and I sincerely believe this book will provide good insight on their way to healthier lifestyles.

To you all, I am so grateful for this process.

Olojo   Christiana.

CHAPTER 1
UNDERSTANDING FAD DIETS

Fad diets have become a hallmark of modern culture, sometimes offering rapid weight loss and usually a shortcut to health. Most fad diets are not backed by scientific evidence and can contribute to a variety of health and other problems. In this chapter we will establish what a fad diet is, describe its characteristics, and then give some historical examples to show you how fads recycle over time.

FAD DIETS-DEFINITION AND CHARACTERISTICS

Fad diets are a genus of dieting plans which promise startling results within a very short period and usually do not require exercise or major lifestyle changes. These diets often gain a following overnight that might link to celebrity endorsements, social media, or other types of virus marketing. They are not easy to be sustained though, and often lead to poor health conditions.

Some Key Characteristics of Fad Diets are:

1. Rapid Result: Fad diets promise rapid results, such as losing 10 pounds in one week. This usually occurs by drastically reducing the calorie intake or by avoiding whole groups of food altogether.

2. Restrictive Nature: Fad diets have a set of rules that one should eat and should not eat. These may include abstaining from carbohydrates, fats, or even a certain group of foods, which will definitely cause deficiencies.

3. Celebrity Endorsements and Marketing Hype: Fad diets are always presented by celebrities or some other influential individual. Thus, it gives them an urgency feeling and attractiveness. The marketing might exaggerate the expected results of the diet.

4. Fleeting Popularity: Fad diets are generally short-lived. When the initial excitement wears off or the side effects start to kick in, interest in the diet begins to fade, and it is usually replaced by another diet that is currently trending.

5. Psychological Appeal: Fad diets are designed to appeal to people's desires for quick fixes and immediate gratification. They promise an easy solution to complex issues relating to weight and health, which in a fast-paced society could be particularly enticing.

6. Risk of Yo-Yo Dieting: Most of the people following fad diets go through a process of losing and gaining weight, thus getting into what is called yo-yo dieting. It is very hazardous for physical and mental health.

HISTORICAL EXAMPLES OF POPULAR FAD DIETS

Fad diets have existed for decades, with many of the same ones surfacing over and over again in different disguises. Here are some historical examples to consider that really outline the trends and pitfalls of fad dieting:

1. The Grapefruit Diet (1930s)

One of the earliest fad diets, the Grapefruit Diet, claimed that one could achieve substantial weight loss by eating grapefruit. The diet prescribed grapefruit or grapefruit juice with every meal because it supposedly contained fat-burning enzymes. While some people did lose weight, the diet was highly restrictive and lacked many nutrients.

2. The Cabbage Soup Diet (1950s)

This diet promised rapid weight loss by consuming a low-calorie cabbage soup for seven days. Participants could eat some fruits and vegetables but were restricted from other foods. While some people do lose weight, this is a diet not sustainable due to nutritional deficiencies.

3. Atkins Diet (1970s)

The Atkins Diet popularized a low-carb type of food which increased the intake of high proteins and fats while drastically reducing carbohydrate consumption. While highly valued at first for its efficiency in losing weight, it also received much criticism concerning health risks it supposedly created in the heart and kidney problems. Controversies notwithstanding, it had several revivals and re-editing along the years.

4. The South Beach Diet (2000s)

This diet, developed by cardiologist Arthur Agatston, is one that allows moderation in a diet of healthy fats and carbohydrates-the so-called South Beach Diet. Very popular at the beginning of its propagation because of its clearly defined stages of development, it also faced criticism for highly restrictive nature and ways unhealthy eating may have been encouraged.

5. Paleo Diet (2010s)

The Paleo Diet advocates for the inclusion of food that was supposedly available to our Paleolithic ancestors; therefore, lean meats, fish, fruits, vegetables, nuts, and seeds, excluding processed foods, grains, and dairy. While it calls for whole foods, critics say it can be overly restrictive and lead to nutrient deficiencies.

6. The Keto Diet (2010s-Present)

The ketogenic diet, or keto diet, has surged in popularity in recent years, emphasizing high fat, moderate protein, and very low carbohydrate intake. While some individuals report weight loss and improved energy levels, the diet can be difficult to maintain and may lead to adverse health effects, such as nutrient deficiencies and increased cholesterol levels.

7. Intermittent Fasting (2010s-Present)

Intermittent fasting has recently been popularized for its weight-loss effect by cycling between periods of eating and fasting. Though there is some evidence of possible health benefits from certain studies, critics warn that the diets may not be right for everyone and may engender unhealthy eating habits.

It is relevant that fad diets be identified with their possible risks and side effects on physical and mental health. By considering their characteristic features and historical examples, we can understand the tendency of diets to recur cyclically and the importance of finding an equilibrium and adopting a proper attitude towards food continuously.

CHAPTER 2
THE SCIENCE BEHIND WEIGHT LOSS

Weight loss, for whatever reason, can be achieved through a science. The chapter discusses the basic principles of weight loss and metabolism, as well as the reasons quick fixes do not work. By understanding these concepts, readers will be better equipped to make informed choices regarding their diet and steer clear of fad diets.

BASIC PRINCIPLES OF WEIGHT LOSS AND METABOLISM

Weight loss basically is all about energy balance, a relationship between the food and beverages calories taken in and the calories expended through physical activities and metabolic processes.

Energy Balance
A. Caloric Intake
This refers to the total number of calories taken in through food and drink. Different foods have different caloric values, determined by their composition of macronutrients-carbohydrates, proteins, and fats.

Energy Expenditure: The total number of calories expended by the body, including:

Basal Metabolic Rate: The number of calories the body needs to maintain basic physiological functions going, even at rest, such as breathing, blood circulation, and cell regeneration. BMR constitutes about 60-75% of total daily energy expenditure.

Physical activity: The amount of calories being burned from types of movement, including exercise and daily activities. It greatly varies depending on a person's lifestyle and activity level.

Thermic effect of food: Energy expenditure for digestion, absorption, and processing of food. This accounts for approximately 10% of the total daily energy expenditure.

Weight Loss Equation: The process of weight loss necessitates one important factor: a caloric deficit. This means that an individual should consume fewer calories than he or she expends. An estimated deficit of some 3,500 calories is normally thought to constitute a loss of about one pound. At the same time, this view is too simplified because individual metabolic rates and body compositions can vary greatly.

B. Metabolism

Metabolism is a set of biochemical processes involved in converting food into energy. Conventionally, metabolism is divided into two categories, namely catabolism and anabolism, wherein energy release and energy consumption by the cell take place, respectively. These will be defined as the breaking down of molecules to derive energy from them and the synthesis of all compounds needed by the cells, respectively. Anabolism would involve the construction of proteins, nucleic acids, and other such important molecules.

Factors affecting metabolism include:

Genetics: Genetic makeup determines one's metabolic rate and the speed at which food is digested in the body.

Age: As a rule, metabolism slows down with age, leading to a reduction in BMR.

Muscle Mass: More calories are burned while at rest in muscle tissue compared to fat tissue; thus, the higher the muscle mass, the more efficient one is at burning calories.

Hormones: Changes in hormone levels in the body affect metabolism, appetite, and fat storage. For instance, thyroid hormones greatly help in regulating metabolic rates.

WHY QUICK FIXES OFTEN FAIL

Despite the attractiveness of quick fixes and fad diets, they usually only bring disappointment and frustration. Knowing the whys behind these failures will make it easier for them to choose better options.

1. Unsustainable Practices

Most of the diets promising quick fixes claim extreme caloric restriction or omission of whole food groups. This may indeed work for some period of time, but usually such practices are not easy to maintain in the long run. Once people return to their usual eating habits, they usually regain the weight they lost in the first place, often resulting in yo-yo dieting.

2. Nutritional Deficiencies

Most fad diets are extremely deficient in one or more of the important nutrients and can lead to deficiency diseases. For instance, a diet devoid of carbohydrates can result in inadequate fiber intake, while diets with low fat can eventually cause deficiencies in essential fatty acids and fat-soluble vitamins. A long-term deficiency in these nutrients contributes to a variety of serious health problems.

3. Metabolic Adaptation

When a person severely cuts down on their food intake, the body can do the opposite and slow its metabolism down to preserve energy. This is called metabolic adaptation, which makes losing weight even harder over time. While the body gets used to using less and less calories, it ends up slowing down the process for the individual, who, out of frustration, may resort to even more extreme measures in an attempt to speed up the process again.

4. Psychological Factors

Quick fixes do not consider the psychological aspects of eating and weight management. Most fad diets put one in a restrictive mindset, which leads to feelings of deprivation and an unhealthy relationship with food. This can result in binge eating or emotional eating, where individuals turn to food for comfort or as a reward. The psychological toll of constant dieting can also lead to anxiety, depression, and a negative body image.

5. Inadequate Education and Support

Many who start on quick-fix diets lack the education and support they need to make a difference in their lives. People are not able to understand principles of nutrition and good eating habits, which may inhibit the ability to maintain weight loss when stopping the diet. Absence of a supportive community is really challenging with which to stay motivated and accountable.

6. Short-Term Focus

Quick fixes generally promote results rather than health and wellness. The promotion of success that is short-term might also cause people to prefer rapid weight loss to the changes in life that can be sustained. On the other hand, an integrated behavior towards eating and exercise offers a healthy attitude towards food and lifelong weight management.

Weight loss as a science is a basis to find one's way through confusions related to dieting and will also give long-lasting results. To understand how energy balance and metabolism work empowers an individual with the choices to be made in order to support health and well-being. Understanding why quick fixes do not work will help the reader find healthier, more effective ways to manage weight.

CHAPTER 3
THE PSYCHOLOGICAL IMPACT OF DIETING

Dieting can be perceived as a very simple approach to attaining one's body weight or shape. On the other hand, the consequences of dieting on one's psychology are serious and far-reaching. This chapter is going to consider how dieting impacts mental health and the link between dieting and disordered eating. Having an understanding of these psychological effects would help readers in living life with regard to their eating habits and maintain a much healthier relationship with food.

HOW DIETING AFFECTS MENTAL HEALTH

Weight loss dieting has massive effects on mental health, which affects emotional well-being, self-esteem, and quality of life. Following are some of the ways dieting influences mental health:

1. Increased Anxiety and Stress

A majority of individuals experience increased anxiety and stress when following a diet. The pressure of having to reach certain weight losses, following strict food rules, and not being able to enjoy "forbidden" foods may make a person anxious all the time. The anxiety can take many dimensions, including obsessive thoughts about food, body image, and weight. The fear of not being able to succeed or achieve results may increase such feelings, thus creating stress and forcing the individual to adapt to unhealthy coping mechanisms.

2. Negative Body Image

Dieting often encourages a narrow definition of beauty and success, which makes individuals develop negative body images. The more an individual compares him/herself to the cultural expectations of what is considered the right body type and the idealized media images, the more dissatisfaction he/she becomes with his/her body. A negative self-concept then sets in, possibly accompanied by feelings of inadequacy, low self-esteem, and depression. The more an individual focuses on weight and appearance, the more likely he or she is to internalize negative beliefs about the self.

3. Emotional Eating and Guilt

Dieting can create a paradoxical relationship with food, in which periods of restraint are immediately followed by periods of indulgence. When people deny themselves foods, they often become preoccupied with a strong wish to eat those foods, which, in turn, can precipitate episodes of emotional eating. This is most often followed by feelings of guilt and shame, hence starting a vicious circle. The emotional power of this cycle can foster stress and anxiety, even more significantly impeding the establishment of a healthy relationship with food.

4. Social Isolation

Dieting can also contribute to social isolation in that an individual avoids social situations that will expose them to food, such as parties, family gatherings, or dining out. The fear of judgment or not being able to keep up with dietary restrictions may make them shy away from social interactions. In effect, this can increase feelings of loneliness and depression, furthering a negative impact on their mental health.

5. Obsessive Behaviors

For some individuals, dieting turns into obsessive preoccupation with intake of food and the execution of exercises. It includes counting of calories, weighing of food items, or extreme amounts of exercises to make atonement for the perceived diet offenses. These behaviors take lots of time and mental energy, which may be used by an individual to focus elsewhere, hence boosting stress and anxiety levels.

THE CONNECTION BETWEEN DIETING AND DISORDERED EATING

The relationship between dieting and disordered eating is intricate and multi-dimensional. While dieting itself does not cause an eating disorder to develop in everyone, a very strong correlation does exist between restrictive dieting practices and the onset of disordered eating behaviors. Key points to consider:

1. Dieting as a Risk Factor

Dieting is a major risk factor in the development of eating disorders among adolescents and young adults. Such restricted eating may trigger an intense interest in food, weight, and body image that leads to disorders such as anorexia nervosa, bulimia nervosa, and binge eating disorder.

2. The Role of Restriction

Restrictive dieting may lead to a vicious cycle of deprivation and bingeing. When individuals severely limit their intake of food, after some time, they may reach a point of overwhelming craving, which could result in episodes of binge eating. The cycle can make a person lose control, feel guilty, and develop shame, which then furthers the disordered eating pattern. The body naturally reacts to restriction by seeking food; this is often overeating when an opportunity arises.

3. Cognitive Distortions

Dieting may create food and body image-related cognitive distortions. In these instances, a person sees all foods as being "good" or "bad." All-or-nothing thinking produces extreme feelings of guilt or shame after consumption of foods believed to be "bad." Guilt or shame often fortifies disturbed patterns of eating. An obsessive focus on weight and body appearance leads to distorted perception of their body shape and structure.

4. The Effect of Media

Social media only increased the connection between dieting and disordered eating. Platforms that idolize body images and diet culture create environments where individuals feel they have to be like unrealistic goals. Exposure to "fitspiration" and diet-related content triggers unhealthy behaviors and negative body image in potentially vulnerable groups.

5. Support and Education

Dieting is, therefore, associated with several untoward psychological effects and may open up the risk for disorders such as anorexia or bulimia. It hence requires a supportive environment, proper education on nutrition and good hygiene, self-acceptance, and healthy coping mechanisms. A health professional, therapist, and support group can help support these individuals in their relation with food and body image in a way that is healthier.

The psychological effects of dieting are far-reaching, and anxiety, depression, and disorders in eating behavior are all possible outcomes for mental health. All these effects have to be understood in the light of developing a better relation with food and body image. By knowing the link between dieting and mental health, a person will be able to make more informed choices as to their eating pattern and will be able to care for themselves much better.

CHAPTER 4
PHYSICAL CONSEQUENCES OF EXTREME DIETING

Extreme dieting often involves severe calorie counting, cutting out whole categories of food, or living on meals and snacks that are nutritionally imbalanced. But despite their appeal to those seeking a quick fix for weight loss or to improve their general appearance, extreme diets hold serious threats to physical health. This chapter will discuss the several health risks of extreme dieting, including nutritional deficiencies and their effects on the body.

SHORT-TERM AND LONG-TERM HEALTH RISKS

Extreme dieting leads to a variety of health concerns. These health concerns can be short-termed or long-term concerns. Understanding these risks becomes of utmost importance in making appropriate dietary decisions.

1. Short-Term Health Risks

The immediate effects of extreme dieting can be shocking and may include:

Fatigue and Weakness: One of the most prevalent short-term effects of extreme dieting is fatigue. Once the body does not get enough calories, it lacks the energy it needs to carry out daily activities. This may lead to feelings of weakness, lethargy, and a decline in physical performance. Individuals may find it difficult to engage in regular exercise or even perform routine tasks.

Dizziness and Lightheadedness: Severe caloric restriction might lead to low blood sugar levels, which can make one suffer from dizziness, lightheadedness, or even fainting spells. This is perilous because this will increase the chances of accidents and injuries.

Digestive Issues: Extreme dieting can impede normal digestion. People can easily become constipated, bloated, or start to have diarrhea because of too little fiber intake or sudden changes in diet. These added digestive problems certainly make one more uncomfortable and ill-pleased with the whole aspect of dieting.

Mood Swings and Irritability: Mood swings and irritability are part of the psychological toll extreme dieting can cause. Prolonged physical hunger, along with nutritional deficiencies and chronic stress associated with adhering to very rigid rules of eating, further creates anxiety and emotional instability.

2. Long-Term Health Risks

The long-term effects of extreme dieting can be more serious and may include:

Metabolic Slowdown: Prolonged calorie reduction can result in metabolic slowdown-the process whereby the body adapts itself to a low caloric intake by decreasing the basal metabolic rate. Resting now, it means the number of calories that the human body would burn at complete rest decreases, resulting in lesser ability to sustain the reduction in body weight and possibility of regaining weight after returning to normal eating habits.

Hormonal Imbalances: Extreme dieting can disrupt the delicate balance of hormones that work together to control hunger, metabolism, and reproductive cycles. For example, an imbalance between leptin-the satiety hormone-and ghrelin-the hunger hormone-leads to increased hunger and cravings. In females, extreme dieting may even cause menstrual disturbance or amenorrhea-the absence of menstruation-which in turn could be much harmful to reproduction in the long run.

Bone Density Loss: Severe caloric restriction combined with inadequate nutrient intake has the adverse effect of bone density loss, which can increase the risk for osteoporosis and fractures. This can be especially alarming for women who, after a certain age, are more prone to problems related to osteoporosis.

Cardiovascular Issues: Extreme dieting has many adverse effects on the cardiovascular system. The quick loss of weight may result in an electrolyte imbalance, increasing the risk of developing arrhythmias and other heartbeat abnormalities. Moreover, loss of lean body mass will have adverse effects on the heart since the heart itself is a muscle that needs nourishment to work properly.

Development of Eating Disorders: Most forms of extreme dieting heighten a person's chance of catching an eating disorder such as anorexia nervosa, bulimia nervosa, or binge eating disorder. The vicious cycle of restraint and bingeing may develop an overall volatile relationship with food and may present serious long-term psychological and physical health consequences.

NUTRITIONAL DEFICIENCIES AND THEIR EFFECTS ON THE BODY

Extreme dieting often results in nutritional deficiencies, which can have serious consequences for overall health. The body requires a variety of nutrients to function optimally, and a lack of these essential components can lead to a range of health issues.

1. Common Nutritional Deficiencies

A. Vitamin Deficiencies

Vitamin D: Essential for bone health and immune function, a deficiency in vitamin D can lead to weakened bones and increased susceptibility to infections.

Vitamin B12: Important for nerve function and the production of red blood cells, a deficiency can lead to anemia, fatigue, and neurological issues.

B. Mineral Deficiencies

Iron: A lack of iron can lead to iron-deficiency anemia, resulting in fatigue, weakness, and impaired cognitive function.

Calcium: Insufficient calcium intake can contribute to decreased bone density and an increased risk of fractures.

C. Macronutrient Deficiencies

Protein: Inadequate protein intake can lead to muscle loss, weakened immune function, and impaired recovery from injuries.

Healthy Fats: A lack of healthy fats can affect hormone production and overall cellular health, as well as lead to deficiencies in fat-soluble vitamins.

2. Effects of Nutritional Deficiencies on the Body

The consequences of nutritional deficiencies can be wide-ranging and severe:

Impaired Immune Function: Nutritional deficiencies can weaken the immune system, making individuals more susceptible to infections and illnesses. A lack of essential vitamins and minerals can impair the body's ability to mount an effective immune response.

Cognitive Decline: Deficiencies in certain nutrients, such as B vitamins and omega-3 fatty acids, can negatively impact cognitive function, leading to issues with memory, concentration, and overall mental clarity.

Skin and Hair Health: Nutritional deficiencies can manifest in skin and hair health. For example, a lack of essential fatty acids can lead to dry skin and hair, while deficiencies in vitamins A and E can result in skin issues such as acne or dermatitis.

Fatigue and Weakness: As mentioned earlier, inadequate nutrient intake can lead to fatigue and weakness, impacting daily functioning and overall quality of life.

The physical consequences of extreme dieting are significant and can have lasting effects on health. From short-term risks such as fatigue and digestive issues to long-term complications like metabolic slowdown and nutritional deficiencies, the dangers of extreme dieting cannot be overstated. Understanding these risks is essential for making informed dietary choices that prioritize overall health and well-being.

CHAPTER 5
THE ROLE OF SOCIAL MEDIA IN DIET CULTURE

Social media is a powerful medium by which perceptions of health, beauty, and body image are being shaped. It brings many opportunities for social connection and community building; on the other hand, it plays a big role in the perpetuation of unattainable body ideals and diet culture. This chapter will look into the way social media has been a contributing factor in the issues associated with unattainable body ideals and social media personalities influencing dietary trends.

HOW SOCIAL MEDIA PROMOTES UNREALISTIC BODY STANDARDS

Social media platforms like Instagram, TikTok, and Facebook have their timelimes flooded with pictures and texts that very often glorify one particular kind of body while creating a narrow definition of what constitutes beautiful. This has serious ramifications regarding how individuals view themselves, perceive their bodies, and develop along paths of mental health.

1. Curated Perfection
Social media allows users to curate their online personas often featuring a snapshot or more accurate representation of an ideal self. Curation could mean:

Filtered Images: Most of the users make use of filters and editing skills to enhance their appearance-smoothening skin, changing body shapes, and even facial features. Such filtered images lead to a false perception of reality among the followers that such appearances are achievable and normal.

Selective Sharing: People tend to share only the best moments and exclude those struggles and imperfections that make one's daily life. It is here where selective sharing creates an environment in which followers feel inadequate with their lives in comparison to other people who seem to be living a perfect life.

2. The Emergence of the "Fitspiration" Culture

The "fitspiration" movement, which promotes fitness and healthy living, can often blur the line between health and appearance. While it may be to inspire others to lead healthier lifestyles, the reality is that many fitspiration posts emphasize aesthetics over well-being. This can manifest in several ways:

Weight Emphasis: Most fitspiration accounts are about weight loss where one is more likely to come across before-and-after shots of a sudden drastic change in body shape. This enforces the idea that self-worth is associated with one's appearance and that drastic measures should be resorted to in order to have a perfect body.

Glorification of Extreme Measures: A number of fitspiration images extol extreme dieting, over-exercise, and other harmful practices for bodies they idolize. Consequently, it has been seen to cause some followers to begin the harmful behaviors in order to attain a fantasy body ideal.

3. Comparison Culture

Social media promotes a comparing culture wherein individuals are measuring themselves constantly against others. This will create:

Negative Body Image: Long-term exposure to idealized imagery may induce feelings of one's personal insufficiencies and low self-esteem. A subject may develop a tendency to view the body as imperfect or deformed, with associated disappointment and unhealthy connotations.

Pressure to Conform: The need to belong and be accepted will make people conform to the expectations within society as regards beauty, at the expense of health. This pressure leads to unhealthy dieting practices, disordered eating, and a preoccupation with weight and appearance.

THE IMPACT OF INFLUENCERS AND DIET TRENDS

Social media influencers are important in the development of diet culture and trends. Their reach and influence have great potential to impact the perception of health and body image in their followers.

1. Influencers as Authority Figures

Most social media influencers present themselves as experts in health, fitness, and nutrition without any professional training or qualifications. This may lead to:

Misinformation: Influencers might promote diets, supplements, or fitness routines that are not evidence-based. In this case, followers might be misled to believe these methods are effective or safe when they may actually be dangerous to their health.

Unrealistic Expectations: Influencers usually post their own transformations, which could set unrealistic expectations for their followers. Assuming immediate results may be achieved, individuals might engage in extreme dieting practices that are neither maintainable nor healthy.

2. Viral Diet Trends

Social media also creates mainstream obsessions with various diet trends-mostly in a way that is completely disrespectful to their safety or viability. Some examples include:

Detox Diets: Most of these diets promise that dieters will lose weight by abstaining from certain foods or by using detox products. These diets lead to nutritional deficiencies and, most of the time, may fail to produce the long-term results a dieter is looking for.

Intermittent Fasting: Some people find it very helpful, but a lot of them misinterpreted it and applied it the wrong way. The influencers promote extreme types of fasting, which leads to eating disorders and other poor conditions of health.

Clean Eating: The clean eating fad implies that some foods are "good" and some foods are "bad." Such polar views on food have been demonstrated to create a bad relationship with food, thereby instigating feelings of guilt and shame toward food consumption.

3. Community and Accountability

While social media can perpetuate harmful diet culture, it can also be a source of community and accountability for some. Supportive online communities can help people share experiences, celebrate successes, and encourage one another in their health journeys. However, these communities should be approached with caution:

Echo Chamber: Online communities can serve as echo chambers where potentially unhealthy beliefs and practices are reinforced. A person may feel obligated to conform to the group's standards, though those standards are not healthy.

Lack of Professional Guidance: Most people use social media for advice on health, rather than seeking professional help. This can lead to misinformation and harmful practices.

Social media plays a multi-approached role in diet culture: on one hand, it might allow unrealistic body standards to be promulgated, even to the extent of supporting the worst kind of diet trends, but on the other, it creates communities and support networks. In such a way, navigating this digital landscape asks people to develop media literacy and critical thinking to distinguish between healthy inspiration and harmfully unsupportive messaging.

CHAPTER 6
DEBUNKING COMMON DIET MYTHS

With diet culture abounding and a myriad of conflicting nutritional information, there are plenty of misconceptions about food and health. These misconceptions can lead to unhealthy eating habits, poor diets, and poor relationships with food. The goal of this chapter is to dispel some of the most common diet myths, including those surrounding calories, carbohydrates, fats, and the truth about detox diets and cleanses.

DEBUNKING COMMON MYTHS ABOUT CALORIES, CARBS, AND FATS

1. Myth: All Calories Are Created Equal

The most ingrained myth within diet culture is that calories do not differ in any way, shape, or form. Such misbeliefs may cause a person to take into consideration only the caloric intake and not the quality of food that is being taken.

A. Quality vs. Quantity

While it is true that weight management is all about balance between consumed calories and calories burnt, the source of those calories makes quite a big difference. For instance:

Nutrient-Dense Foods: Fruits, vegetables, whole grains, lean proteins, and healthy fats provide one with necessary nutrients that keep good health going. These foods usually give one a feeling of satiety, that is, they keep the stomach full for a longer time to avoid overeating.

Empty Calories: In contrast, foods with added sugars and unhealthy fats, like snacks containing sugar, beverages, and processed foods, offer less nutritional value. These "empty calories" can lead to weight gain and health problems without offering what the body requires.

B. Metabolic Effect

The body has different metabolic modes depending on the nutrient or macronutrient in question.

TEF: is the energy the body uses to digest, absorb, and metabolize food. A greater amount of energy is required to process proteins in comparison with carbohydrates and fats; hence, foods containing high levels of protein will have a higher thermic effect.

Hormonal Response: Various foods can trigger a different hormonal effect regarding hunger and satisfaction. Foods with high sugar might create sharp ups and downs in the level of blood sugar, thereby triggering hunger and cravings.

2. Myth: Carbohydrates Are Bad for You

Carbohydrates have for a long time been demonized in diet culture, with many thinking they are the number one enemy in causing weight gain and health problems. Such a myth simplifies the role of carbohydrates in the diet and utterly disregards the question of quality and quantity.

A. The Role of Carbohydrates

Carbohydrates are the major source of energy for the body, and this is especially true for the brain and the muscles. They are important for:

Physical Activity: Carbohydrates provide the fuel needed for exercise and daily activities. Athletes and active individuals require adequate carbohydrate intake to maintain performance and recovery.

Nutritional Benefits: Most foods rich in carbohydrates, such as fruits, vegetables, legumes, and whole grains, are powerhouses of vitamins, minerals, and fiber. These nutrients are indispensable in maintaining general health and can even help prevent chronic diseases.

B. Complex vs. Simple Carbohydrates

Not all carbohydrates are created equally. But first, it is important to understand the difference between what is called complex and simple carbohydrates:

Complex Carbohydrates: These are found in whole grains, legumes, and starchy vegetables, which digest slowly, providing a steady release of energy and satiety.

Simple Carbohydrates: These are found in sugary foods and beverages; simple carbohydrates are digested very fast, hence causing a rapid rise in blood sugar levels. Though they may give fast energy, their excessive consumption leads to gaining weight and health problems.

3. Myth: Fats Make You Fat

Much like carbohydrates, dietary fats have been villainized in popular diet culture. The notion that eating fat makes one gain weight is a myth that ignores the diversity of dietary fats and their relationship with health.

A. The Importance of Healthy Fats

Fats are needed for a number of bodily functions, including:

Hormone Production: Fats are required for the synthesis of hormones, which include but are not limited to sex hormones and metabolic hormones.

Nutrient Absorption: Some vitamins, notably vitamins A, D, E, and K, are fat-soluble, and their proper absorption in the body depends on their intake with dietary fat. Healthy fats can, therefore, increase the nutritional value of a meal.

B. Types of Fats

Knowing the types of fats will help in making informed choices in diets:

Unsaturated Fats: These are considered heart-healthy and help with the reduction of inflammation. Foods rich in unsaturated fat include items such as avocados, nuts, seeds, and olive oil.

Saturated Fats: Although some saturated fats, for example, in coconut oil and dairy products, can be part of a healthy diet, overconsumption of saturated fats coming from processed foods may lead to health problems.

Trans Fats: These are bad fats that are usually found in foods with a lot of preservatives and fried foods, which increase the risk for heart diseases.

THE TRUTH ABOUT DETOX DIETS AND CLEANSING

Detox diets and cleansing have become popular over the years and have been promoted as ways to lose weight and be healthy quickly. However, most of these practices involve myths and can lead to harm to the body.

1. Myth: Detox Diets Are Necessary for Health

A very common myth is that the body needs help to "detoxify" itself. The human body is fully capable of detoxification by itself through its organs like the liver, kidneys, and digestive system.

The Body's Natural Detoxification

Liver Function: The liver metabolizes the toxins and removes them from the body. The liver processes nutrients and filters out harmful substances, keeping the body balanced and healthy.

Kidney Function: The kidneys filter out waste products from the blood and excrete them through urine, helping to maintain fluid and electrolyte balance.

Digestive System: A healthy digestive system is helpful in eliminating waste and toxins by way of regular bowel movements.

2. Myth: Cleanses Cause Permanent Weight Loss

Most detox diets and cleanses boast of rapid weight loss, sometimes by drastically reducing calorie intake or omitting whole categories of nutrients. These results are usually temporary and may have adverse effects on health.

Temporary Weight Loss

Water Weight: In most cases, the weight shed in the initial stages of any cleansing diet is actually just a loss of water weight, not fat. This can often create a sense of false satisfaction that can easily turn into disappointment if the weight is regained shortly after returning to normal patterns of eating.

Extreme calorie restriction can cause muscle loss that would be detrimental to metabolism and health in general.

Detox Dieting

Many detox diets are very low in essential nutrients, leading to nutrient deficiencies and generally affecting health. Prolonged intake of such diets can be characterized by the following:

Fatigue and Weakness: Generally, when one does not consume enough calories and nutrients, this might make one feel very weak and tired and may render an individual unable to attend to daily activities.

Impaired Immune Function: Generally, malnutrition lowers the body's immunity, thus being highly prone to diseases and infections.

3. The Psychological Consequences of Detox Diets

The consequences of detox diets are not only physical but also psychological, such as the following:

Guilt and Shame: The nature of a detox diet will breed guilt and shame with regards to food, hence an unhealthy relationship with eating.

Yo-Yo Dieting: These extreme restrictions and then binge eating build on one another, leading to yo-yo dieting, or what many refer to as weight cycling.

Now that it is time to debunk the diet myths, this can help in forming a very healthy relationship between food and body image. Knowing how complex calories, carbohydrates, and fats can be will similarly make people more aware of their dietary choices and not fall prey to the pitfalls of diet culture..

CHAPTER 7
THE CYCLE OF YO-YO DIETING

Yo-yo dieting, or weight cycling, refers to the alternation of body weight loss and regaining, usually caused by extreme methods of dieting. Such a process may be quite frustrating and dejecting for an individual looking ahead to a healthy weight level. Understanding the mechanisms of yo-yo dieting, besides the physiological and psychological effects, is of primary importance in order to be able to break out of such a destructive pattern. This chapter examines the cycle of weight loss and regain, looking at various effects that yo-yo dieting has on the body and mind.

UNDERSTANDING THE CYCLE OF WEIGHT LOSS AND REGAIN

Yo-yo dieting typically starts when an individual initiates a diet in hopes of losing weight quickly. The yo-yo diet can be divided into several key phases:

1. Starting a Diet

People often start diets for losing weight as quickly as possible. This can be manifested by:

Extreme Caloric Restriction: Most diets allow only a drastic caloric deficit to make one lose weight very fast at least for some time. The problem is, they are hard to keep up and usually create a sense of deprivation.

Food Group Elimination: Certain diets advise completely eliminating a particular food group, such as carbohydrates or fats. This will make one develop an unhealthy relationship with food and give in more to cravings.

2. Initial Weight Loss

Most people lose weight during the initial stages of dieting because of the following reasons:

Water Weight Loss: Oftentimes, the body will relinquish water weight at the beginning of a diet. These quick results can be encouraging.

Fat Loss: Over time, as one increasingly restricts their calories, they will most likely start losing fat. The lost fat, however, is normally coupled with muscle loss, which inversely affects metabolism.

3. Plateau and Frustration

As the diet progresses, individuals may encounter a weight loss plateau, where further weight loss becomes challenging. This can lead to:

Increased Hunger and Cravings: Prolonged caloric restriction can trigger hormonal changes that increase hunger and cravings, making it difficult to adhere to the diet.

Psychological Stress: The frustration of not seeing continued results can lead to feelings of disappointment and stress, prompting individuals to abandon their diet.

4. Relapse to Old Eating Habits

After the abandonment of diet, people usually go back to their old eating habits; these include:

Binge Eating: The circle of restriction gives way to binge eating periods whereby one takes in volumes of food within a short time. Usually brought about by feelings of deprivation, it's accompanied by guilt and shame.

Weight Regain: When individuals go back to their previous habits, the lost weight is regained, and in many cases, they may put on even more weight than before, and hence the starting point for another diet is higher.

5. Repeat Cycle

It can also be a self-repeated cycle where individuals keep on trying quick fixes for losing weight. This can result in a range of negative consequences, from physical to psychological.

THE PHYSIOLOGICAL AND PSYCHOLOGICAL EFFECTS OF YO-YO DIETING

The effects of yo-yo dieting transcend mere fluctuations in weight. Physiological and psychological effects both can have long-lasting consequences for a person's health and general well-being.

1. Physiological Effects

A. Metabolic Adaptation

The largest quantity of physiological effects, related to yo-yo dieting, pertains to metabolic adaptation. This implies that one's body adjusts itself against a lesser intake of calories:

> *Decreased Basal Metabolic Rate:* The result of this recurrent weight loss and subsequent gain is a decrease in the BMR-the amount of calories the body needs to burn per day, while resting. This will make subsequent attempts to diet much harder to do.

> *Loss of Muscle Mass:* Severe diets are often associated with loss of muscle, which again contributes to the lowering of metabolic rates. Muscle tissue is metabolically active and requires more calories than fat tissues. The loss of muscle actually impedes weight loss and encourages fat accumulation.

B. Hormonal Imbalances

Yo-yo dieting can disturb the balance of hormones that help in regulating appetite and metabolism:

> *Leptin and Ghrelin:* Leptin is that hormone which gives the signal of satiety, while ghrelin stimulates appetite. Repeated rounds of weight loss and regain ultimately lead to lower levels of leptin and

higher levels of ghrelin, leading to increased hunger and cravings.

Insulin Resistance: Changes in weight also contribute to insulin resistance, in which the body shows lesser sensitivity to insulin. This would therefore heighten the chance of suffering from type 2 diabetes and other metabolic syndromes.

C. Increased Fat Storage

The body could respond to episodes of food scarcity by adopting better fat-storing strategies:

Changes in Fat Cells: The repeated weight cycling may increase the number and size of fat cells, making it easier to gain weight after dieting. It's a vicious circle: the more one diets, the harder it becomes over time to lose weight.

2. Psychological Effects

The psychological effects of yo-yo dieting can be far-reaching and complex:

A. Body Image Issues

These constant weight fluctuations have a very negative effect on body image and satisfaction:

Self-esteem: People may feel insufficient and develop low self-confidence by comparing themselves to standards of beauty set in society. This could result in obsession with weight and appearance.

Disordered Eating Patterns: This might promote the beginning of some kind of eating disorder, including binge eating disorder or orthorexia (obsession with healthy eating).

B. Emotional Distress

Yo-yo dieting has been found to precipitate emotional turmoil and mental health issues:

Anxiety and Depression: The stress associated with constant dieting, and a sense of failure with each regained pound, can affect anxiety and depression. Individuals might feel they are involved in some sort of vicious cycle trying to diet without an apparent exit.

Food Obsession: The emphasis on weight loss and dieting cultivates an unhealthy obsession with food whereby individuals are constantly thinking about what they can and cannot eat. This will develop a very toxic relationship with food and inhibit the ability to enjoy a meal.

3. Breaking the Cycle

The first step to breaking the yo-yo dieting cycle is recognizing its detriments. Some strategies toward a healthier relationship with food and body image include:

Balanced Approach: Instead of extreme dieting, individuals can focus on balanced, sustainable eating patterns that emphasize whole foods and moderation.

Mindful Eating: A person can work out better relations with food through practicing mindful eating, whereby the cues of the body for food-in and food-out are learned to be listened to.

Looking for Professional Help: A registered dietitian or a mental health professional will go a long way in trying to bring about changes in disordered eating habits and devise ways one may deal with nutrition and health.

The yo-yo diet cycle is a very complex and dramatic phenomenon, which may be followed by physiological and psychological long-term impacts. The mechanisms of weight loss and regain, along with the identification of the impacts of the cycle, are necessary toward the breaking free from non-healthy dieting behavior.

CHAPTER 8
THE IMPORTANCE OF MINDFUL EATING

Mindful eating has emerged as a potent antidote to unhealthy dieting habits and disordered patterns of eating. Mindful eating promotes awareness and presence at mealtimes as a means of rebuilding a healthier relationship with food and enhancing overall well-being. This chapter will review what mindful eating is, how it can help, and some practical techniques for developing a more mindful approach to eating.

WHAT IS MINDFUL EATING AND HOW IT CAN HELP

1. Defining Mindful Eating

Mindful eating is a practice based on the principles of mindfulness: paying attention to the moment without judgment. This applied to eating encourages the following in a person:

Being Present: Eating mindfully involves paying attention to the experience of eating food-flavors, textures, aromas-and physical sensations of hunger and fullness.

Attune to Your Body: it allows the individual to hear one's body signals for hunger or being filled, thus helping to feed themselves instead of responding to external foods' availability or emotional eating

Mindfulness on Food: It creates awareness into personal thoughts and feelings towards certain kinds of food. The purpose is to find patterns linked to emotional eating or non-sense snacking.

2. Benefits of Mindful Eating

Mindful eating has a number of benefits that can positively affect one's physical and mental health. These include:

A. Improved Digestion

By slowing down and savoring each bite, individuals can improve digestion:

Chewing Thoroughly: Mindful eating encourages thorough chewing, which aids in the breakdown of food and promotes better nutrient absorption.

Reduced Overeating: Eating slowly allows the body to signal fullness more effectively, reducing the likelihood of overeating and promoting a healthier weight.

B. Enhanced Enjoyment of Food

Mindful eating nurtures greater appreciation for food:

Savoring Flavors: By focusing on the sensory experience of eating, individuals can enjoy the flavors and textures of their meals, leading to greater satisfaction and fulfillment.

Breaking the Guilt Cycle: It allows for the enjoyment of all foods without feelings of guilt. Thus, mindful eating promotes a balanced nutrition approach, where indulgence itself may be part of the path to a healthy lifestyle.

C. Emotional Awareness

With mindful eating, there is increased awareness about one's emotional relationship to food:

Identifying Triggers: By paying attention to thoughts and feelings during meals, individuals can identify emotional triggers that lead to overeating or unhealthy food choices.

Developing Coping Strategies: Mindful eating can help individuals find alternative coping mechanisms for emotional distress, reducing reliance on food for comfort.

D. Weight Management

Research has shown that mindful eating can be a support for weight management efforts:

Sustainable Changes: It is by cultivating a better relationship with food that individuals can create changes in the way they eat to ensure healthier long-term well-being.

Reduce Cravings: Through mindful eating, one learns to observe their hunger and satiation signals, and hence they can make food choices more harmoniously.

TECHNIQUES FOR DEVELOPING A HEALTHIER RELATIONSHIP WITH FOOD

Developing a mindful eating practice requires intention and effort. Here are several techniques to help individuals cultivate a healthier relationship with food:

1. Create a Mindful Eating Environment

The environment in which you eat can significantly impact your eating experience. To promote mindfulness, consider the following:

Minimize Distractions: Turn off screens, put away phones, and create a calm atmosphere during meals. This allows you to focus solely on the act of eating.

Set the Table: Take the time to set the table and present your food attractively. This can enhance your appreciation for the meal and encourage a more mindful approach.

2. Practice Gratitude

Incorporating gratitude into your eating routine can foster a positive mindset:

Reflect on Your Food: Before eating, take a moment to appreciate the food on your plate. Consider where it came from, the effort that went into preparing it, and the nourishment it provides.

Express Gratitude: Whether through a silent acknowledgment or a spoken word, expressing gratitude for your meal can enhance your connection to food and promote a sense of mindfulness.

3. Engage Your Senses

To fully experience your meal, engage all your senses:

Observe the Food: Take a moment to look at your food. Notice the colors, shapes, and presentation. This visual engagement can enhance your appreciation for the meal.

Savor the Flavors: As you eat, focus on the flavors and textures of each bite. Chew slowly and allow the tastes to linger on your palate, enhancing your enjoyment of the meal.

4. Tune into Hunger and Satiety Cues

Listening to your body's signals is a cornerstone of mindful eating:

Assess Hunger Levels: Before eating, take a moment to assess your hunger level on a scale from 1 to 10. This can help you determine whether you are truly hungry or eating out of habit or emotion.

Pause During Meals: Throughout your meal, pause periodically to check in with your body. Ask yourself if you are still hungry or if you are beginning to feel full. This practice can help you avoid overeating.

5. Practice Mindful Portion Control

Mindful eating encourages individuals to be aware of portion sizes without strict restrictions:

Serve Smaller Portions: Start with smaller portions on your plate.

You can always go back for more if you are still hungry, but this approach can help prevent overeating.

Use Smaller Plates: Using smaller plates can create the illusion of a fuller plate, helping to satisfy visual cues of fullness while promoting portion control.

6. Reflect on Your Eating Experience

After meals, take a moment to reflect on your eating experience:

Journal Your Thoughts: Consider keeping a food journal where you can write about your meals, feelings, and any insights gained during the eating process. This can help you identify patterns and areas for improvement.

Evaluate Your Satisfaction: Reflect on how satisfied you felt after the meal. Did you enjoy the food? Were you able to listen to your body's cues? This reflection can help reinforce mindful eating habits.

Mindful eating is a transformative practice that can help individuals break free from the cycle of unhealthy dieting and develop a more positive relationship with food. By cultivating awareness, savoring each bite, and tuning into the body's signals, individuals can enhance their enjoyment of meals, improve digestion, and promote overall well-being.

CHAPTER 9
SUSTAINABLE WEIGHT MANAGEMENT

In a society often touting quick fixes and rapid weight loss, few discuss the notion of sustainable weight management. The concept of sustainable weight management is actually about attaining and maintaining a healthy weight through nutritionally balanced diets, regular physical activity, and lifestyle changes that one can maintain over the long haul. This chapter discusses various techniques and methods of maintaining long-term weight with no extreme dieting while incorporating the most essential variables that are necessary in achieving that goal-balanced nutrition and physical activity.

LONG-TERM WEIGHT MANAGEMENT STRATEGIES WITHOUT EXTREME DIETING

1. Realistic Goals

Having realistic and achievable goals is one of the founding concepts in sustainable weight management:

Focus on Gradual Change: A weight loss of 1 to 2 pounds a week is considered a healthy, sustainable rate. These amounts allow for less dramatic lifestyle changes and minimal stress associated with aggressive diets.

SMART Goals: The SMART criteria help set specific, measurable, achievable, relevant, and time-bound objectives. Instead of saying, "I want to lose weight," for instance, a more articulated goal would be, "I will lose 10 pounds in three months by exercising three times a week and eating more fruits and vegetables."

2. Adopt a Balanced Approach to Nutrition

Sustainable weight management rests on balanced nutrition that emphasizes variety and moderation:

Emphasize Whole Foods: Focus on adding whole, minimally processed foods to your diet, including fruits, vegetables, whole grains, lean proteins, and healthy fats. These foods are nutrient-dense and can help you feel full while providing essential vitamins and minerals.

Practice Portion Control: Learn to recognize appropriate portion sizes and listen to your body's hunger and fullness cues. Using smaller plates and serving sizes can help you avoid overeating while still enjoying your favorite foods.

Incorporate Flexibility: Allow for occasional indulgences without guilt. A sustainable approach to eating does include flexibility, which enables treats to be enjoyed in moderation, helping to prevent feelings of deprivation that may lead to binge eating.

3. Develop Healthy Eating Habits

Creating healthy eating habits is essential for long-term success:

Meal Planning and Preparation: Plan your meals and snacks in advance to ensure you have healthy options readily available. Preparing meals at home allows you to control ingredients and portion sizes, making it easier to stick to your nutrition goals.

Mindful Eating As will be discussed in the chapter on nutrition, mindful eating may help you redevelop a healthier relationship with food. By paying attention to your meal and focusing on flavors, smells, textures, and colors, you may find more satisfaction in eating and have less of a tendency to overeat.

Hydrate Your Body: Drinking enough water throughout the day is important to keep your body healthy and also helps in controlling hunger. Sometimes, thirst is disguised as hunger, which results in unnecessary snacking.

4. Incorporate Regular Physical Activity

Physical activity is an integral part of effective weight management:

Activities You Enjoy: Find physical activities that you really enjoy, such as dancing, hiking, swimming, or playing a sport. You are more likely to continue an activity if you enjoy it.

Be consistent and not intense. The key to weight management is consistency. Aim for at least 150 minutes of moderate-intensity aerobic activity or at least twice a week strength training exercises.

Incorporate Movement into Daily Life: Try to find opportunities to be active throughout your day. This can include walking or biking instead of driving, taking the stairs instead of the elevator, or engaging in active hobbies.

5. Monitor Progress and Adjust as Needed

Regularly monitoring your progress can help you stay accountable and make necessary adjustments:

Food and Activity Journal: By recording food and exercise intake, one is able to garner a deeper understanding of one's patterns and how those can be improved. Sometimes this practice reinforces positive behavior and keeps a person on track.

Be Flexible: Weight management is a nonlinear process. Ups and downs come your way, and one needs to be flexible to make necessary changes in strategies whenever needed. If there is a plateau or regain, reassess your goals and make the necessary adjustments to your routine.

THE ROLE OF BALANCED NUTRITION

AND PHYSICAL ACTIVITY

1. Balanced Nutrition

Balanced nutrition is the backbone of sustainable weight management. Eating a wide variety of foods in order to get all the nutrients your body needs for good functioning includes:

A. Macronutrients

The contribution of carbohydrates, proteins, and fats to weight reduction must be understood to implement a correct diet.

> *Carbohydrates:* These are the primary source of energy. Focus on complex carbohydrates: whole grains, fruits, and vegetables, supplying fiber and necessary nutrients.

> *Protein:* Protein is vital to the building and repair of muscle and further may even minimize appetite. Lean protein needs to come from poultry, fish, legumes, tofu, and low-fat dairy.

> *Fats:* Good fats are important in making hormones and in the absorptive process of nutrients. Add sources of unsaturated fat, like avocados, nuts, seeds, and olive oil, limiting saturated and trans fats.

B. Micronutrients

Micronutrients, which include vitamins and minerals, are important for good health: Variety is Key Eating a rainbow of different colored fruits and vegetables will provide you with a range of different vitamins and minerals. Aim for a minimum of five servings of fruits and vegetables each day.

Consider supplements in addition if necessary. It may be easier to get many nutrients from whole foods instead of supplements, but they help with some dietary restrictions. Seek the advice of a qualified physician to do so.

2. Physical Activity

Physical activities are essential not only as an aspect of weight but more so in general health:

A. Benefits of Doing Regular Exercise

There is numerous advantages of regular exercising:

Weight Management: Exercise burns calories, creates a calorie deficit condition-the effect responsible for losing weight-and maintains muscles when one is on dieting. This is important since one's metabolic rate decreases as muscle mass decreases.

Improve Mood and Mental Outlook: Endorphins are emitted when one engages in exercise that alleviates and reduces symptoms of depression, leading to improved mood. Increased exercise can also improve sleeping capabilities as it allows one to have heightened self-esteem.

Improved Cardiovascular Health: The heart is strengthened through regular aerobic exercise, improving circulation and reducing the risk of heart disease and other chronic conditions.

B. Integrating Physical Activity into Daily Life

There are ways to make the inclusion of physical activity in daily life more feasible:

Active Transportation: When possible, walk or bike to work or take public transportation that involves walking to and from stops.

Break Up Sedentary Time: With a desk job, get up every hour to stand, stretch, or take a short walk. This can help minimize the negative effects of prolonged sitting.

Engage in Family Activities: Engage your family and friends in activities that include physical activity, such as hiking, playing sports, or taking dance classes together. This is a good way to address physical activity and social connection.

The balance between nutrition, physical activity, and other elements of healthy lifestyle habits holds the key to sustaining weight. Setting realistic goals, adopting a balanced diet, incorporating regular exercise, and monitoring progress are ways to create a sustainable framework for long-term success.

CHAPTER 10
THE INFLUENCE OF DIET CULTURE ON BODY IMAGE

Dieting has permeated into daily contemporary society and shapes perceptions of our sense of self-worth, health, and ideas of beauty. This ever-pressuring culture manages to make one central message abundantly clear: thin equates with success, happiness, and desirability. Many today have developed unhealthy attitudes toward diets with the purpose of idealizing their bodies. During this chapter, we will cover how society shapes our perceptions in relationship to body image, followed by reviewing research examining the influence of dieting upon self-esteem and body satisfaction.

HOW SOCIETAL PRESSURES SHAPE OUR PERCEPTIONS OF BODY IMAGE

1. The Role of Media and Advertising

The media plays an enormous role in the creation of general attitudes towards beauty and body shape:

Unrealistic Patterns of Beauty: Advertisements, television shows, movies, and social media often portray only images of thin and conventionally good-looking people. These photos and pictures are normally photo-shopped and filtered, hence distorting reality even further.

Promotion of Dieting and Weight Loss: Media portray the concept of dieting as the only way to succeed in being beautiful. Everywhere, advertisements on weight loss products, fad diets, and cosmetic surgery support the idea that one should strive for an aspired body type to gain acceptance.

2. Cultural Norms and Values

Cultural influences also make their presence felt in perceptions regarding body image:

Cultural Ideals of Thinness: In many Western societies, thinness is equated far too often with health, discipline, and self-control. Such a cultural ideal can only result in perpetuating in individuals self-worth tied to body size, hence leading to feelings of worthlessness and dissatisfaction.

Intersectionality and Body Image: Different cultures have different beauty ideals, and individuals from marginalized communities face increased pressures to adhere to the dominant culture's beauty standards. Such intersectionality can exacerbate body image issues as individuals navigate confusing messages regarding their culture, beauty, and self-worth.

3. Social Media Influence

The rise of social media has increased the effects of diet culture on body image:

Comparing Culture: Social media encourages comparison. People will be led to take a closer look at their bodies compared to the pictures of curated images from influencers and other people. Comparing tends to bring in dissatisfaction with oneself.

Curated Lives: Most people on social media portray a high version of themselves, including filtered photos and edited videos. This curated reality creates unrealistic standards of body image and lifestyle that may cause envy or low self-esteem in viewers.

4. Peer Pressure and Social Expectations

Pressure from one's peers and social networks could have an immense influence on body image:

Conformity to Group Norms: The social groups one belongs to may pressurize individuals to adhere to the body ideals of the group through unhealthy dieting behaviors, which lead to body dissatisfaction. This is especially pronounced in adolescents and young adults when they are most susceptible to peer influence.

Body Shaming and Bullying: Negative remarks from peers concerning body size or appearance have long-term effects on self-esteem and body image. More often, body shaming leads into a vicious circle of dieting and disordered eating as one aims to fulfill the expectations in society.

THE IMPACT OF DIETING ON SELF-ESTEEM AND BODY SATISFACTION

1. The Psychological Effects of Dieting
Dieting has powerful psychological consequences beyond those that relate to physical appearance.

A. Increased Body Dissatisfaction

Temporary Results: Weight loss achieved through dieting is usually temporary; the individual regains the weight after a certain period, leading to disappointment and a feeling of failure. Such loss and regain in a cyclical manner can make the individuals suffer from body dissatisfaction and poor self-concept.

Focus on Appearance: Dieting often shifts the focus from overall health and well-being to appearance and weight. This emphasis on looks may result in a distorted body image, where individuals become overly critical of their bodies and less appreciative of their overall health.

B. Heightened Anxiety and Depression

Emotional Distress: The pressure to be perceived as beautiful might heighten anxiety and depression. Individuals may experience being overwhelmed by the nonstop pursuit of an ideal body, leading to feelings of inadequacy and hopelessness.

Disordered Eating Patterns: These are the eating behaviors prompted by dieting, including binge-eating, restrictive eating, and obsessive calorie counting. The behaviors then contribute to mental health problems and serve to create a negative feedback loop of body dissatisfaction and emotional distress.

2. Self-Esteem and Body Image

Self-esteem and body image are closely intertwined, and the practice of dieting may have a profound effect on both:

A. Self-Worth Tied to Appearance

Conditional Self-Esteem: People link self-esteem with appearance; they believe that one will be valued or accepted only for acquiring a particular body size or shape. The result of such conditional self-esteem is that it may lead to a never-ending circle of dieting and disappointment.

Social Validation: In the case of gaining acceptance, one can resort to extreme ways of dieting; to be accepted by society becomes the greatest drive. External acceptance builds self-worth so precarious that negative comments and any fluctuation in weight become cause for disarray.

B. Positive Body Image and Self-Esteem

Developing a Positive Relationship with One's Body: A positive body image involves the understanding and appreciation of the body as being functional rather than just something to look at. This shift in thought may enhance self-esteem and contribute to overall well-being.

Self-compassion: Self-compassion is an attitude that may help individuals handle the challenges of body image with understanding and kindness. By offering oneself the same amount of compassion as one would offer a friend, one will be able to establish a healthier relationship with their body and reduce the harmful effects of dieting on self-esteem.

3. Breaking the Diet Culture Cycle

Diet culture can bring negative impacts on body image, and for that, one needs to take active control:

Challenge Societal Norms: Recognize and confront the unrealistic expectations of beauty set by society. Surround yourself with diverse depictions of beauty; engage in media that celebrates body positivity and inclusivity.

Focus on Health, Not Weight: Shift the focus away from weight loss and to health and well-being. Emphasize feeding the body with balanced nutrition, and participating in physical activities that are enjoyable rather than punitive in nature.

Seek Support: Avail yourself of supportive communities that foster body positivity and self-acceptance. Connecting with others who have had similar experiences, through social media, support groups, or therapy, helps build resilience against diet culture pressures.

Diet culture powerfully and pervasively influences body image, building perceptions of beauty and self-worth in ways that can be harmful to both mental and physical health. It is within such an understanding of societal pressures toward body dissatisfaction and recognition of the self-esteem effects of dieting that individuals are empowered to better take care of themselves toward a healthier relationship with their bodies.

CHAPTER 11
NAVIGATING DIETARY RESTRICTIONS AND PREFERENCES

With dietary choices now being dictated by health conditions, ethical considerations, and personal preferences, the navigation of dietary restrictions can be rather daunting. From medical conditions ranging from diabetes to food allergies, or mere lifestyle choices like vegetarianism and veganism, being prepared for these diets means knowledge that is paramount for health and well-being. This chapter shall outline and discuss best practices in the management of dietary restrictions due to health conditions and personalized nutrition for optimal health outcomes.

DIETARY RESTRICTIONS FOR HEALTH CONDITIONS: HOW TO APPROACH THEM

1. Dietary Considerations for Common Health Conditions

There are some health conditions that require special diets, which help in alleviating the symptoms and improving the health condition. Following are some of the more common conditions and considerations regarding their diets:

A. Diabetes

Management of diabetes involves critical planning regarding carbohydrate intake and general nutrition:

Carbohydrate Counting: People with diabetes often find that learning to count carbs is a good way to work toward blood sugar stability. Foods containing carbohydrates have different effects on blood glucose.

Glycemic Index: Foods with a low GI will be digested slowly and result in a gradual increase in the level of blood sugar. Incorporating low-GI foods, such as whole grains, legumes, and non-starchy vegetables, can contribute toward managing blood sugar.

Balance in Meals: Emphasize balanced meals that include a mix of carbohydrates, proteins, and healthy fats to help stabilize blood sugar levels and prevent overeating.

B. Food Allergies and Intolerances

Food allergies and intolerance necessitate the strict avoidance of certain foods to halt adverse reactions:

Identifying Triggers: The first line of management in food allergies involves the identification and elimination of the precipitating foods. Common allergens include nuts, dairy, gluten, soy, and shellfish.

Reading Labels: Food allergic individuals should be good at reading labels for the allergens hidden. That means being aware of terminology indicating possible allergens and situations for cross-contamination.

Substitutions: It is very vital to find suitable alternatives to these allergenic foods. The person with lactose intolerance could switch to lactose-free products in their usual dairy or switch over to plant-based ones.

C. Celiac Disease

The onset of celiac disease is mediated through an immune response against gluten; thus, the treatment consists of a strict gluten-free diet. That means avoiding all sources of gluten, including wheat, barley, and rye. Gluten-free grains include quinoa, rice, and buckwheat.

Cross-Contamination Awareness: A person has to be fully aware of cross-contamination during food preparation and intake. It involves the usage of different utensils and cooking surfaces to avoid exposure to gluten.

2. Consulting Healthcare Professionals

In the case of diet management regarding health issues, consulting a health professional is highly necessary:

Registered Dietitian: A registered dietitian will offer personalized nutrition recommendations based on individual health needs. They will be able to help create meal plans, educate about food choices, and give strategies for managing dietary restrictions.

Medical Guidance: Certain conditions, such as diabetes or celiac disease, require regular check-ups with healthcare providers to monitor health status and make dietary adjustments as necessary.

THE IMPORTANCE OF PERSONALIZED NUTRITION

1. Understanding Personalized Nutrition

Personal nutrition is truly a unique science in that dietary needs and preferences can vary greatly from one individual to another. Some factors that would influence personalized nutrition include:

Genetics

Genetic predisposition will affect how individuals metabolize nutrients, react to certain foods, and their vulnerability to specific health conditions. Understanding these genetic factors informs dietary choices.

Lifestyle Factors: The lifestyle a person lives, including activity, stress, sleep, and work environment, is hugely important in determining nutritional needs. Such factors are considered in personalized nutrition to make dietary recommendations based on specific cases.

Cultural and Ethical Considerations: Food choices are highly influenced by one's cultural background and ethical beliefs. Personalized nutrition respects the culture and values of the client, which in turn enables the individual to follow preferences yet maintain proper nutrition.

2. Benefits of Personalized Nutrition

There are several advantages of personalized nutrition in relation to general diet plans.

A. Improved Health Outcomes

Targeted Nutritional Interventions: With personalized nutrition, nutritional interventions become more specific for the improvement of certain health outcomes. For example, a patient with high cholesterol may be counseled on a diet rich in omega-3 fatty acids and soluble fiber.

Improved Compliance: When dietary recommendations align with the individual's preference and lifestyle, one is likely to follow the prescription. In such a case, long-term health goals are achieved.

B. Increased Awareness and Education

Empowerment through Knowledge: Personalized nutrition encourages individuals to learn about their bodies and how different foods affect their health. Knowledge empowers an individual to make informed choices about diet.

Skill Building: Most personalized nutrition encompasses teaching about meal planning, cooking skills, and label reading to enable the patient to interact in their diet optimally.

3. Delivery of Personalized Nutrition

Delivery of personalized nutrition may be achieved by considering the following steps:

A. Individual Need Assessment

Complete Evaluation: Conduct a thorough assessment of eating patterns, health status, lifestyle factors, and personal preferences in cooperation with a dietitian or nutritionist.

Goal Identification: Clearly establish realistic goals pertinent to the individual's needs and preference. The goals may revolve around weight management, an energy boost, or effective control of some health condition.

B. Designing a Meal Plan Individualized

Personalized Meal Plans: Create a meal plan that comprises a wide variety of foods, keeping in mind the restrictions and preferences. The focus should be on nutrient-dense foods that can deliver the body's requirement of vitamins and minerals.

4. Flexibility and Adaptability

The meal plan needs to be flexible and adaptable. Life changes, cravings, and social pressure will surely cause one to make changes, and it is here one should consider a personalized approach to dieting.

Regular Check-ins: Regularly set check-ins to measure progress and make necessary changes in the meal plan. This may be as simple as tracking food, monitoring health markers, or just talking about challenges.

Feedback Loop: Encourage open dialogue around what is working and what isn't. This feedback loop will keep the diet continually evolving to be both effective and enjoyable.

The need to navigate food restrictions and preferences is highly complex in nature-it calls for a lot of understanding, flexibility, and personalized ways of handling. Recognizing the particular diets related to health conditions and embracing the power of personalized nutrition will lead to improved health outcomes and overall better well-being.

CHAPTER 12
FINDING SUPPORT AND RESOURCES

The journey to healthier eating and sustainable weight management is fraught with barriers in a culture so saturated with competing dietary messages and quick fixes. Finding the right kind of support and resources is so crucial in navigating these very challenges. This chapter will explore the vital role that healthcare professionals play in guiding healthy eating and emphasize how support groups and communities are a big help for those who have trouble dieting.

THE ROLE OF HEALTH PROFESSIONALS IN GUIDING HEALTHY EATING

1. Understanding the Expertise of Health Professionals

Health professionals who are responsible in guiding eating healthily and resolving dietary concerns include registered dietitians, nutritionists, physicians, and mental health specialists. These provide the following services:

A. Registered Dietitians

Personalized Nutrition Counseling: RDs are trained to offer nutrition counseling that is individualized for the specific health needs, dietary preference, and lifestyle of a person. They will be able to help one come up with a personalized meal plan that will keep one healthy.

Evidence-Based Guidance: RDs apply evidence-based practices in educating clients about nutrition. They continually update themselves on the latest research and current dietary guidelines to make sure recommendations are based on scientific evidence.

Management of Health Conditions: RDs, especially for individuals who have specific health conditions like diabetes, heart disease, or food allergies, can recommend special diets that will manage symptoms and improve overall health.

B. Physicians

Comprehensive Health Assessments: Physicians can provide comprehensive health assessments to identify any underlying medical conditions that may impact dietary choices. They can also order necessary tests to monitor health markers, such as cholesterol levels or blood sugar.

Referrals to Specialists: Physicians can refer patients to registered dietitians or nutritionists for specialized dietary guidance. This collaborative approach ensures that patients receive comprehensive care tailored to their needs.

C. Mental Health Professionals

Overcoming Emotional Eating: Emotional eating may be effectively approached and overcome with the help of mental health professionals, like psychologists and counselors, through the instigation of healthier relations with food. They can provide coping mechanisms to deal with stress, anxiety, and body image concerns.

Support for Disordered Eating: Mental health professionals can extend therapy and support when individuals are suffering from disordered eating behaviors and help them overcome these problems in order to eventually have a much healthier attitude toward food.

2. How to Access Healthcare Support

Finding the right healthcare support involves the following steps:

A. Identifying Your Needs

Evaluate your needs: Define what you're trying to achieve with nutritional change: whether it be weight, energy, or another health-related issue; knowing your goals will help lead you to the right person.

Consider Your Preference: Consider whether you prefer a registered dietitian, physician, or a mental health specialist. Each professional differs in style; it's pertinent that you find one whose style relates to you.

B. How to Research Professionals

Seek recommendations. Get recommendations from your friends, family members, and health providers. Sometimes these personal referrals can result in finding professionals who have track records.

Check their credentials, find RDs or licensed nutritionists qualified by education and training in this field.

Review: See the online reviews and testimonies; people's reviews could give a peek into one professional's capabilities and attitudes that others could have hired him for consultation. c. Scheduling of Consultation

Initial Consultation: Most of these practitioners offer initial consultations, whereby one can discuss needs and set goals. Utilize the opportunity to question their modality, experience, and how they can best serve you.

Assess for Compatibility: If comfortable and understood by the professional, this is an assurance of a good rapport necessary in effective collaboration.

SUPPORT GROUPS AND COMMUNITIES FOR THOSE STRUGGLING WITH DIETING

1. Strengths of Community Support

The support groups and communities can be crucial to any individual with diet problems for the reasons described below.

A. Shared Experience

Connection to People: Support groups create channels through which one individual could get to meet others with almost identical problems. This shared struggle dispels loneliness and opens up free expressions and sharing of troubles or experiences.

Learning from Peers: Hearing the different journeys that others experience is bound to bring new insights and how diets can be best managed coupled with health goals. The participants have lots to share: tips on practical recipes, mechanisms for managing such conditions.

B. Psychological Support

Comfort of Understanding: Support groups at times offer psychological support from an understanding perspective. Members can encourage each other forward when success is achieved or during disappointing outcomes.

Accountability: A supportive community often fostakes accountability. This is achieved through regular check-ins and discussions of each other's progress.

2. Types of Support Groups and Communities

There exist several types of support groups or communities for individuals who go through dieting challenges, including:

A. In-Person Support Groups

Local Community Centers: Most community centers and health institutions offer a support group in a physical environment dealing with nutrition, weight management, and eating healthy. These are excellent groups since there is always a structured environment where discussions and learning occur.

Health Clinics: Other healthcare clinics also engage patients with particular health conditions into support groups, such as diabetes or eating disorder groups. Such groups may be moderated by healthcare professionals and become sources of great information.

B. Online Support Communities

Social Media Groups: Several groups on Facebook and Instagram focus on eating healthy, managing weight, and loving your body. The spaces created can offer the same sense of support and inspiration coming from many different people.

Website/Forums: Sites like Reddit and MyFitnessPal have pages and online forums where one could share experiences, ask questions, and look for advice on others with similar experiences.

C. Weight Loss Programs

Structured Programs: Most weight loss programs, such as Weight Watchers or Noom, include group meetings and online communities. These programs will offer structured support, meal planning resources, and accountability via group interactions.

Workshops and Classes: Local health organizations or local fitness centers may offer workshops and classes focused on nutrition education, cooking skills, and making healthy lifestyle changes. Such settings foster community and practical skill-building.

3. How to Find and Join Support Groups

Finding the right support group includes some steps:

A. Research Available Options

Online Searches: First of all, search online for support groups in your area or an online community that suits your needs. The use of keywords regarding one's diet or health issues will help in the search.

Ask for Recommendations: Approach your doctor, friends, and family for advice on good support groups or communities.

B. Evaluate Group Dynamics

Group Size and Structure: Observe the size and composition of the group. Small groups can provide more individualized attention, while larger groups provide a wider range of experiences.

Facilitator Qualifications: If a facilitator leads the group, research their qualifications and level of experience. A well-versed facilitator can elevate the effectiveness of the group through valuable insights and guidance.

C. Participate Actively

Join the Group: Once found, join the support group and actively participate in the discussions and activities it holds. You will be further enriched by sharing your story and helping others.

Set Goals with the Group: You may want to work with other members of the group to set a common goal or challenge. This might be one more way to build camaraderie and encourage one another.

It takes support and resources to navigate all the different diets, their restrictions, and food preferences. Medical professionals are a great source of guidance and expertise, while support groups and communities can provide psychological encouragement through sharing experiences. In such a way, resources will enable people to work toward getting a healthier relationship with food for better well-being and reaching their health goals..

CHAPTER 13
REDEFINING HEALTH AND WELLNESS

The society tends to equate thinness with health; the definition of health and wellness is in dire need of revision. Conventional thinking-a focus on weight above all else-leads to diets that can be very destructive, resulting in an unhealthy relationship between food and one's body image. This chapter discusses the importance of moving beyond weight as a measure of health while emphasizing the importance of holistic well-being and self-acceptance in leading a healthier and more balanced life.

MOVING BEYOND WEIGHT AS A MEASURE OF HEALTH

1. The Limitations of Weight as a Health Indicator

Traditionally, weight has been used primarily as a measure of health; however, there are several limitations to this approach:

A. Body Composition vs. Body Weight

Understanding Body Composition: Body weight is not a full indicator of a person's health. The proportion of fat, muscle, bone, and water that makes up a person's body gives a more correct definition of health. He or she may weigh more due to the increase in muscular mass, which is healthier.

Health at Every Size: This approach embraces the fact that a person, irrespective of body weight or size, can strive toward being healthy and well. On a whole new dimension, the emphasis here is that health may not be judged based solely on weight parameters.

B. Weight Stigma

Weight Bias and Discrimination: Putting emphasis on weight as an indicator of health only worsens the stigma of weight and discrimination. Individuals with larger bodies are often judged even within health facilities, which may lead to poorer care and consequently poor health outcomes because of that stigma. This could even discourage people from attending medical consultations or developing healthy habits.

Psychological Consequences: The pressure to conform to cultural standards of weight brings anxiety, depression, and disturbed eating. When a person relates self-esteem to weight, it is like setting up a cycle that fosters negative body image and harmful dieting practices.

2. Alternative Measures of Health

To redefine health, there is a need to consider the various measures that encompass a more holistic concept of well-being. Such alternative measures include:

A. Physical Health Indicators

Body Mass Index/Blood Pressure/Cholesterol: Each of these parameters regarding blood pressure, cholesterol level, and heart rate variability seems uninfluenced by body weight for diagnosis of cardiovascular health.

Blood sugar levels, insulin sensitivity, and inflammation markers constitute critical variables of metabolic health; and these are assessed on account of routine blood tests alone - events or practices that may be absolutely independent of the influence of body weight variations.

B. Psychological/Emerotional Well-being

Mental Health Assessments: Psychological well-being is part of health. Regular mental health assessments, including screening for anxiety and depression, may yield a full picture of the well-being of a person.

Stress Management: The ability to manage stress effectively is critical for overall health. Mindfulness, meditation, and yoga practices enhance mental resilience and contribute to a healthier lifestyle.

C. Functional Health

Physical Activity Levels Assessment: The ability to conduct physical activities such as walking, climbing stairs, or sports will give insight into functional health. Regardless of weight, regular physical activity is associated with numerous health benefits.

Quality of Life: Quality of life measures, including satisfaction with life, social connections, and overall happiness, are critical indicators of well-being. These factors contribute to a holistic understanding of health that goes beyond weight.

EMPHASIZING HOLISTIC WELL-BEING AND SELF-ACCEPTANCE

1. The Concept of Holistic Well-Being

Holistic well-being encompasses multiple dimensions of health including physical, mental, emotional, social, and spiritual:

A. Physical Well-being

Nourishing the Body: Approaching the body as something one nourishes rather than looking to diet to achieve bodily ideals can be an effective promoter of physical health. Eating a variety of whole foods will lead to a balanced diet consisting of fruits, vegetables, whole grains, lean proteins, and healthy fats.

Regular Exercise: The most important thing concerning physical health is to exercise regularly; this includes activities one finds appealing and can sustain over a long period, such as walking, dancing, swimming, or whatever kind of movement one enjoys.

B. Mental and Emotional Health

Mindfulness and Self-Care: Being more mindful and practicing self-care methods would help improve one's mental and emotional condition. These are stress-releasing methods, such as meditation, journaling, and time in nature.

Therapeutic Support: Professional help in the form of mental health support will enable a person to deal with emotional issues and come out with better ways of dealing with problems. It provides means for building self-acceptance and resilience.

C. Social Connections

Building Relationships: Good social relationships are very important for emotional well-being. Interacting with supportive friends, family, and communities will provide a sense of belonging and improve general well-being.

Community involvement: Through engagement in community activities or volunteering adds meaning to the individual and contributes to whole person health.

2. Importance of Self-Acceptance

Self-acceptance is another important contributor to the holistic well-being concept that also reinterprets health:

A. Acceptance of body image

Challenging the Norms: Embracing body positivity is going against societal norms and refusing to be held by the thought that self-worth is equated with good looks. The shift in mind helps people learn to appreciate what their bodies can do rather than how they look.

Affirmations and Positive Self-Talk: Positive self-talk and affirmations may help in developing a kinder relationship with one's body. This may include recognizing strengths, celebrating successes, and appreciating beauty in diversity.

B. Resilience Promotion

Building Coping Skills: In building resilience, one needs to learn how to cope with life's difficulties. This will involve learning to handle stress, setting realistic goals, and seeking help where necessary.

Embracing Imperfection: Realizing perfection is not achievable, and it's okay to have imperfections, allows for more self-acceptance. This will help in developing a better relationship with food and body image, without pressuring oneself to live up to unrealistic expectations.

3. Practical Strategies for Redefining Health and Wellness

In embracing a holistic approach to health and wellness, the following strategies may be considered:

A. Setting Holistic Health Goals

Holistic Goal Setting: Instead of focusing on weight loss alone, set goals for holistic health that include various features of health. This can include goals about physical activity, mental health, social connections, and self-care practices.

Celebrate Success: Acknowledge and celebrate progress in all areas of health, not just those to do with weight. Recognizing improvements in mental well-being, energy levels, or social engagement can reinforce positive behaviors.

B. Nurture a Supportive Environment

Surround Yourself with Positivity: Create an environment that supports your holistic health journey. This may involve spending time with positive influences, engaging in uplifting activities, and curating social media feeds that promote body positivity and self-acceptance.

Seek Out Resources: Avail yourself of resources like books, podcasts, and workshops on holistic health and self-acceptance. Exposure to various perspectives will enrich your understanding and maybe even inspire change.

C. Practice Mindful Eating

Listen to Your Body: Engage in mindful eating by encouraging yourself to listen to your body for its own cues about hunger and fullness. This can create a much healthier relationship with food and promote intuitive eating.

Savor the Experience: Allow yourself time to enjoy your meals, appreciating flavors, textures, and nourishment. This might help in increasing the feeling of satisfaction from food, thereby minimizing emotional eating.

A redefined view of health and wellness means a shift in the way people think, transcending weight as an indicator of health. It is only through the holistic approach of being physically, mentally, emotionally, and socially fit that a life of balance can be built. The development of self-acceptance is directly related to body positivity and thus includes a deep appreciation for the body and concentration on general well-being..

CHAPTER 14
EMBRACING A BALANCED
APPROACH TO EATING

In a world drenched by diet fads, quick fixes, and nutritional advice that often conflicts, the ability to adopt a balanced approach to eating is crucial in developing a healthy relationship with food. This chapter summarizes some of the key take-home messages from our journey into the world of unhealthy dieting and invites readers to adopt a more balanced view of food and dieting. This allows them to shift the focus from a restrictive eating pattern to an inclusive, flexible one that will give way to a sustainable lifestyle and overall well-being.

SUMMARIZING KEY TAKEAWAYS

1. The Dangers of Fad Diets and Quick Fixes

Quick Fixes: Fad diets promise fast weight loss and rapid fixes, usually short-lived. These can cause a yo-yo effect where the weight lost is gained again, many times with extra pounds added.

Nutritional Deficiencies: Most of these fad diets forbid one kind of food completely or rely on drastically cutting down on calories. This results in nutritional deficiencies, which influence a person's physical health, energy level, and well-being.

Psychological Consequences: The pressure of meeting beauty demands and obsessive preoccupation with weight loss have disordered eating behaviors, anxiety, and body image disturbances as their common outcomes. For some individuals, the psychological aspects have even become more distressing compared with the physical results of an unhealthy diet.

2. Why Nutritional Requirements Must be Individualized

Individual Needs: Nutrition is not a 'one-size-fits-all' approach. Genetic variability, lifestyle, health condition, and personal preference play major roles in deciding one's nutritional needs. Personalized nutrition thus respects these differences and allows for dietary recommendations accordingly.

Holistic Health: A balanced relationship with food is about physical health, but also mental and emotional. Such a holistic perspective invites one to move beyond obsession with weight and shift focus toward overall wellness.

3. Redefining Health and Wellness

Beyond Weight: Health cannot be defined by body weight or the way the body looks. Health can be envisioned as being physically fit, having proper mental health, emotional stability, and social connectedness. Emphasis on such dimensions allows more holistic notions of well-being.

Self-acceptance: Self-acceptance and body positivity can play an important role in building a healthy relationship with food. Realizing that everybody is different and every human body should be respected empowers the individual to take care of his health without pressuring himself or herself into the ideal which society enforces.

4. Mindful and Intuitive Eating

Listening to the body: Mindful eating and intuitive eating practices allow one to listen to the body and its signals of hunger and satiety.

This attitude toward food helps one enjoy a meal without any guilt or bingeing.

Savor: Taking time to savor and appreciate food can also enhance the eating experience. Mindful eating promotes enjoyment and satisfaction, reducing the likelihood of emotional eating and mindless snacking.

5. Building an Enabling Environment

Community and Connection: Surrounding yourself with supportive people and communities can help in increasing motivation and accountability. Engaging others who share similar goals creates a sense of belonging and encourages positive behaviors.

Access to Resources: Tapping into resources, including registered dietitians, nutritionists, and support groups, offers great opportunities to receive guidance and encouragement on this journey toward balanced eating.

ENCOURAGING READERS TO ADOPT A HEALTHIER, MORE BALANCED PERSPECTIVE ON FOOD AND DIETING

1. Shift Your Mindset

Embrace Flexibility: A balanced relationship to food allows for flexibility and variety. Instead of living by rules, focus on adding a plethora of foods that nourish your body and bring joy. This can help reduce feelings of deprivation and foster a much healthier relationship with food.

Practice self-compassion: Be kind to your journey. Everyone has those moments of indulgence or makes less-than-ideal food choices. Instead of negative self-talk, practice self-compassion and realize health is a lifelong journey and not a destination.

2. Create a Positive Food Environment

Stock Your Kitchen Wisely: Fill your kitchen with a variety of healthy foods you really like. Having healthier options at your fingertips can help you make balanced choices and reduce the temptation to fall back on processed or other less healthy snacks.

Mindful Meal Planning: A way to go about meal planning could be to plan meals that balance macronutrients-carbohydrates, proteins, and fats-along with micronutrients-vitamins and minerals. This way, one is able to feed the body well while enjoying the process of cooking and eating.

3. Joyful Movement

Activities You Enjoy: Physical activity should not be a punishment; it should be enjoyed. So find what works for you, whether that is dancing, hiking, swimming, or yoga. Joyful movement improves physical health and enhances mental well-being.

Listen to Your Body: Pay attention to how your body feels during and after physical activity. This awareness can help you choose activities that energize and invigorate you, rather than those that leave you feeling drained or exhausted.

4. Practice Mindfulness While Eating

Slow Down: Give yourself the time to eat slowly, so you can taste your food. Turn the television off and put away your cell phone. This will give you more time to enjoy your food and a sense of satiety.

Reflect on Your Choices: After the meals, take a moment to reflect how the food really made you feel. Consider whether it satisfied your hunger, and if you enjoyed flavors and textures. This reflection can help you become more thoughtful about your food choices.

5. Get Support and Resources

Connect with Professionals: If you are feeling overwhelmed by all of your dietary decisions, find a registered dietitian or nutritionist who will be able to offer guidance and support specific to your needs.

Supportive Communities: Connect with communities promoting body positivity, intuitive eating, and overall health. Such spaces will foster encouragement, inspiration, and connection on your journey to balanced eating.

The journey toward a balanced approach to eating is one of change in perspective, acceptance of oneself, and holistic well-being. Moving beyond restrictive dieting practices and embracing nourishment, joy, and flexibility in the eating process will help an individual establish a healthier relationship with food and their body. Let this be the takeaway from this journey into unhealthy dieting and the path to wellness: health is not a number on the scale but the richness of your experiences, the joy of nourishing your body, and the love you cultivate for yourself.

BOOK REVIEW

Dear Reader,

Let me seize this opportunity to express my deepest gratitude to each and every one of you for sparing your time to read my book, **"EAT OR BE EATEN**: *"Between The Hidden Dangers of Fad Diets and Quick Fixes"* I am so grateful for your support, and I sincerely hope that the ideas and strategies shared in this book have inspired you in your fundraising activities.

Share Your Thoughts!

If you enjoyed the book, I'd love it if you could take a moment to leave a star review. Your review helps me both as an author to improve, and other readers to find the book. Here's how to leave a review:

1. Head to the store where you bought the book.
2. Find the review section.
3. Rate the book and leave a comment!

Whether it be a few words about what you learned or how the book inspired you, every review counts!

If you enjoyed **"EAT OR BE EATEN,"** I invite you to explore my other books. Each is crafted with the same passion and dedication to the delivery of insight and useful advice as you have found here. Some of my other works you may want to consider:

- [THE BOLD & BANKABLE FEMINIST]
Amazon Book Link: https://www.amazon.com/dp/B0DNTM9QF1

- **[WOMEN'S WORLD OF MONEY]**
Amazon Book Link: https://www.amazon.com/dp/B0DNRC5G5F

- **[THE FINANCIAL ACTIVIST'S BLUEPRINT]**
Amazon Book Link: https://www.amazon.com/dp/B0DNWNRXSC

- **[FROM YOUR SHADOW]**
Amazon Book Link: https://www.amazon.com/dp/B0DP2Z1G2B

- **[THE HIDDEN BATTLE OF GIFTEDNESS]**
Amazon Book Link: https://www.amazon.com/dp/B0DPDN566N

- **[THE INNER WORLD OF CHILDREN]**
Amazon Book Link: https://www.amazon.com/dp/B0DP97Q3LN

- **[LENDING A HELPING HAND]**
Amazon Book Link: https://www.amazon.com/dp/B0DP7DKL17

- **[ESCAPING YOUR HEALTH KILLER]**
Amazon Book Link: https://www.amazon.com/dp/B0DPCGMD8G

- **[EVERY FUNDRAISER]**
Amazon Book Link: https://www.amazon.com/dp/B0DPPNRNHC

- **[BECAUSE 1'M FAT]**
Amazon Book Link: https://www.amazon.com/dp/B0DPS8K47R

You can locate all my books by searching for Olojo Christiana on Amazon with the links above.

Your Support Is Important

Your review and recommendations are of great importance to me in growing my readership, and this will enable me to continue writing. Thank you once again for your support.

Best regards,

Olojo Christiana

ABOUT THE AUTHOR

Olojo Christiana is a passionate health advocate, nutrition enthusiast, and author dedicated to empowering people in making informed choices concerning their diets and ways of life. With a nutritional science background and years of working experience in the wellness industry, Christiana has seen for herself how lives have been torn apart by fad diets and quick fixes.

She does this through her writing: to demystify the complexities of nutrition and provide practical guidance for those seeking sustainable health solutions. As Christiana says, the right approach to eating is based on knowledge and mindfulness, and herein lies the secret to lasting wellness.

In addition to writing, Olojo enjoys cooking healthy meals, trying out new cuisines, and sharing those experiences in workshops and community events. She lives with her family in a home that focuses on healthy lifestyles and wholeness.

Connect with Olojo Christiana by buying and reviewing all her book on Amazon.